On the evening of August 25, 2017, my life changed on a surgical table at a hospital in Dallas, Texas. My life had inexplicably crossed paths with a beautiful young lady, aged 39 years, by the name of Joni Marie.

Joni Marie had checked the box. The box of life.

When she became an organ donor, Joni Marie had no idea that she would be extending the life of someone who was five years her senior.

Someone who had battled Cystic Fibrosis for 44 years. Someone who was at the point where this disease was attempting to finish its sole and barbarous mission of destroying a life.

Someone whose lung function was at 17%. Someone whose doctor said he would not live beyond the end of that year without a lung transplant.

Joni Marie became my hero. My knight who rode in on that mythical white horse in her shining armor. The one who saved my life.

Joni Marie was and is my angel donor.

I dedicate the stories in this book to Joni Marie. The person to whom I owe my life.

I also dedicate these stories to her parents, Beverly and Kenneth. The ones who raised Joni Marie to be the giving and loving daughter, sister and mother she became. The ones who taught her the values and principles that ultimately led her to the unselfish decision to become an organ donor.

The ones who influenced her to develop the mindset that ultimately saved my life.

Thank you for taking the time to read these stories, and to share in this journey which Joni Marie has enabled me to undertake and to live.

If these stories touch you as much as they touch me, please write a review about this book to let me know. I would love to hear about your journey.

Rod Spadinger

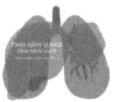

Table of Contents

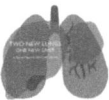

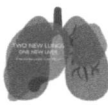

#1 – September 1, 2018

At the age of 44, I received a double lung and liver transplant a week before I turned 45. I wasn't anxious about the surgery. I didn't think it would really happen, I didn't think it would work, I didn't think I needed it. A year later, I found that I was wrong on all points. It happened, it worked, and I needed it.

#2 – September 2, 2018

It's one of those times when I think about how it is to breathe through someone else's lungs. It's kind of unsettling, if one were to spend too much time doing so, I have to admit. The thought that it's possible to pull someone's organs out of their body, and place it smack dab into someone else's. Do that for a pair of lungs, then for a liver. Amazing.

Not long ago, that would have been just science fiction-type fantasy. It makes you wonder what tomorrow might bring.

#3 – September 3, 2018

I'm about to head out for a day trip. It's a holiday, so there's no better time.

New lungs, so there are no coughing fits at stoplights. Not having coughing fits going along at 60 mph, trying to find one of the several napkins stored in the car door, while keeping at least one hand on the wheel at all times, looking straight ahead. That maneuver has to be just as risky as attempting to find a dropped cell phone under your brake pedal. :)

At any rate, off I go. Have a great day!

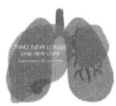

#4 – September 4, 2018

(*O*)ne of the priceless benefits I was provided with this transplant I received last year is that I am able to enjoy new experiences and learn new stories. Please allow me to share one of those amazing experiences and stories from yesterday.

Yesterday, I took a drive from Dallas, TX to my mom's hometown in Kansas. It was one of the most amazing journeys I have ever taken.

I started talking to an elderly man outside of a Conoco gas station about a cane he was using. As it turns out, this random person I ran into remembers my mother's family, and that they had many children. He remembers my mother's brother, my uncle.

To make the encounter even more unique, when I told him yesterday that I was taking pictures of the town because her birthday was the following day, on September 4th. He then told me that he was born on September 3rd (which was, of course, yesterday) - of the same year! He was born a day before her. So even though he didn't remember my mom, given the small town where they lived, this man and my mom had to have been classmates.

Imagine that! I go to Humboldt, Kansas, to visit my mom's hometown, and I begin a conversation with a stranger who turned out to have been one of her classmates.

And one last irony in this story - this man's birthday is September 3rd. My birthday is also September 3rd. He and I shared a birthday yesterday.

No words to explain this happenstance, but it's just one more reason I am thankful that my donor allowed me a second chance in life.

#5 – September 6, 2018

(*Y*)esterday, I read a post from someone who also has Cystic Fibrosis. It brought back all sorts of memories. This young lady commented about how she is soon to begin a round of home IVs, despite her performing regular respiratory treatments, in hopes of warding off the

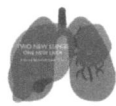

bacteria that persistently festers and fosters itself in her lungs, as a CF patient.

She discussed how the home IVs would be a two-week treatment, potentially to be extended if her lung functions did not return to baseline. About her concern that insurance may be combative due to her current out of state treatment status. About her thoughts regarding the side effects of the antibiotics whose intended purpose are to kill destructive bacteria, but they are also perceivers in destroying healthy bacteria as well, resulting in uncomfortable consequences the patient must deal with while endeavoring to heal from the lung infection. Reading this lady's post left a knot in my stomach. It brought me directly back to those same times I and all CF patients must endure periodically and regularly.

This is even more of a reason to thank my donor for the gifts she provided me. For her generosity. At the same time, I hope and wish that each CF patient suffering will be connected to the type of generous person to whom I became connected. The one who checked the box. Who checked the box to give me a second chance.

#6 – September 8, 2018

A few days ago, someone who is nice enough to follow this blog mentioned that perhaps these postings may reach those who currently are registered to donate their organs. I would be thrilled and honored if I could be a part of that course of understanding.

Given that Cystic Fibrosis is a genetic disease, I was born with this ailment. I have always been aware that CF would likely result in an early demise, and since approximately 10 years ago, I knew that a lung transplant could be an option to extend my life. All the same, for a variety of reasons, I did not consider that procedure to be something I wanted to undertake.

So, when I checked the box on my driver's license so many years back, I did so without a thought of the great benefit it could provide a person. I had no idea of the tremendous impact it can have on the lives

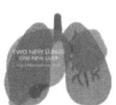

of the recipients. Further, I did not know how much good one donor could do for so many people, and in so many ways. I simply checked the box.

Prior to my experience, I thought all that could be donated were organs – a heart, lungs, liver and kidneys. I now know much differently. I had no idea about tissue donations, let alone the impact they can have on the recipients.

According to the Donate Life website, donated tissue such as skin, bone, and heart valves can dramatically improve the quality of life for recipients, and help save lives, including saving patients with severe burns, allowing athletes with torn ligaments or tendons to heal and regain strength, restoring hope and mobility to military men and women who have been injured in combat, and repairing musculoskeletal structures such as teeth, skin, and spinal components.

Each year, approximately 39,000 tissue donors provide lifesaving and healing tissue for transplant. Approximately 1.75 million tissue transplants are performed each year. One donor's cornea could restore sight to two people. One donor's tissue can heal the lives of 75 people.

If you are not already, please consider becoming an organ donor. As of 2:28 pm EST today, there are 74,873 individuals who are active waiting list candidates. One person is added to the national transplant waiting list every ten minutes, and twenty-two people die every day while awaiting a transplant. Eight thousand deaths occur each year in the U.S. because organs are not donated in time.

One donor can save eight lives and affect the lives of countless others. Every life saved creates a story for that person rescued. Take the opportunity to create eight stories.

#7 – September 10, 2018

Not long after I received the transplants last August, I was told that I would be able to contact my donor's family a year after the surgery to thank them. That would be my opportunity to communicate my gratitude, to find out about my donor, who she was, what she was,

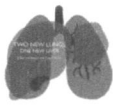

and to whom. I told myself that I would begin drafting that letter immediately, editing it as time went on, so that when the one-year mark came about, the letter would be ready.

However, I found it more difficult than I expected to begin to compose the letter. How do you approach a family who you don't know? How do you reach out to people who have lost their loved one, while here I am alive with great health? Enjoying life now that the Cystic Fibrosis I've had my entire time barely affects me. While the number of holidays I will experience have been extended exponentially, their holidays will be forever minus one.

After much thought, the letter is now written, and has been sent. Even though the words are there in text, expressing my sincere appreciation for their loved one and her sacrifice is unable to be communicated in mere words.

To meet the family, to show my thanks in an embrace, in a handshake, is something I dearly look forward to.

#8 – September 12, 2018

I was at a doctor's appointment the other day. As part of the typical tests during the appointment, the oxygen saturation level in my blood was measured. The meter read 100%.

100%.

Those with Cystic Fibrosis have a sense of nervousness, of apprehension, much or little, of what that reading will show. The better the number will mean that the next IV treatment, the next hospitalization, will not be recommended this time.

100%

On the other hand, a lower number comes with the concern that you might be admitted following this visit. Or if not this visit, perhaps soon enough. Then the thoughts go through the mind of whether this is a dark trend. It leads to questions of when the numbers will improve. Or to the thought of whether it will ever improve.

100%

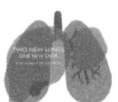

That figure is more than just three numbers followed by a symbol. There is a meaning to that measurement. 100% for someone who has Cystic Fibrosis is not just unattainable. It is much bigger than that. It is a sign of life. It is a sign of hope. It is a sign that you are okay, that you are going to be okay.

100%

Prior to my transplant, my oxygen saturation was at 17%. But as a result of my donor's gift, this time, the reading was at 100%.

#9 – September 16, 2018

A few weeks back, Allison Holt, a young lady with Cystic Fibrosis who had a relatively recent lung transplant, passed away. Of course, when anyone leaves us, it is absolutely tragic, but this one seemed more impactful to me.

Although I did not know this beautiful person very well, as I regrettably only knew her through Facebook, I felt a type of connection with her. When I found that she had passed, I read through her recent posts in an attempt to learn more about her journey that was cut short far too soon. I learned that she received her transplant at approximately the same time I did. Likely in the same month.

As much as it made me sad to know that her second chance was so awfully short-lived, it made me think about the game of drawing straws. I remember using that game when I was young as a method of deciding who would win whatever contest was at hand. The one who drew the longest straw won the contest. I always considered that to the be the lucky straw. Or conversely, the one who drew the shortest straw lost the game. That was the unlucky straw.

In this instance of the lung transplant scenario occurring in the same month, one could say that Allison and I played a game. We drew straws. I have profoundly mixed feelings about the results of that game between us. I am extremely fortunate and thankful to be doing very well with my health a year post transplant. Allison, I am moved deeply to say, is no longer with us.

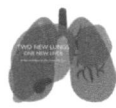

In this game, in this instance, I drew the lucky straw. Allison drew the unlucky straw. I won the game. I won the contest. Allison did not.

Not a day passes when I do not wonder how I drew the lucky straw. Not a day passes when I wonder how the winner of this contest is ultimately decided. How it is determined who pulls the lucky straw, and who doesn't. I will wonder this each and every day of my life.

Truly. I will.

#10 – September 19, 2018

Hope is an emotion that can serve as a powerful tool. Hope is what gets us up in the morning. Hope that it will be a good day at work. Hope that it will be an enjoyable day off. Hope is what we consider as we end the day. Hope that tomorrow will be a good day, and maybe better than the one that just ended.

It is that same hope which supports and encourages those who are sick. Hope that they will heal and be better after a certain period of time. As with all patients who have Cystic Fibrosis, I went through many bouts of sickness, many hospital visits, many treatments with home IVs. During those several decades of treatments, including both daily maintenance at home and those described above, there was the hope that although there was certainly no cure on the horizon, or even a largely effective treatment available, I would be able to move onto the next day of my life. Onto my next adventure. And so forth.

Regrettably, it is entirely likely that there will be a time when a CF patient faces the reality that it is possible, regardless of how many treatments the person has had, it will not be enough to sustain them.

I came to that point a couple of years back. Despite my condition and 17% lung function, I did not feel as if I needed a transplant. I was convinced that I could successfully continue down the path of increasing hospital visits, which wound up mandating longer hospital stays, and use my oxygen compressor infrequently, and only when I absolutely had to. Even though I could no longer shop, since pushing a grocery cart made me short of breath and somewhat light-headed, I was able

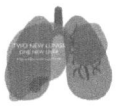

to rely on grocery delivery services to my apartment. Online shopping sufficed for other goods of which I was in need. So, I thought I would be fine without any excessive intervention.

All the same, in the back of my mind, I knew that a transplant might be an option for me. Even though I did not think a transplant would be effective, I was aware that if I did succumb to the reality of accepting someone else's organs someday, there would be the hope that I might make it to the end, and in a positive manner.

As fate dictated, it was late in the day, late in the month of August 2017, that this hope became a reality for me, thanks to my beautiful donor. If she had not checked that box at some point in the past, perhaps some place as ordinary as a DMV, perhaps when she was in the presence of a loved one who is now grieving for her loss, as a mere afterthought, or performed due to a deep commitment to the cause, who knows which end I would have been dealt.

Hope is a precious commodity. Each and every person who volunteers to be an organ donor adds one more light, one more beam, to that ray of hope. Because my donor chose to add a little more brightness to that beam, to that ray, I am here to type this portion of my story this evening.

Forever grateful.

#11 – September 22, 2018

After an organ transplant, the patient is prescribed a number of medications, a number of pills. Some of the pills are vitamins and that sort, but most are anti-rejection drugs. Throughout the patient's life, the body will attempt to reject the transplanted organ, as it sees this object from a different person as foreign. Part of the routine of managing the level and amount of the medication involves the patient undergoing blood tests.

Generally, the amount and type of medications prescribed for the patient immediately post-transplant are at a routine drug type and dosage. But during the weeks and months subsequent to the transplant,

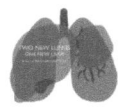

the patient's blood is analyzed to find the optimal level of medication, with the dosage of the meds, and sometimes even the meds themselves, adjusted accordingly. If the medication dosage is too high, it could lead to a toxic level of the drug in the bloodstream. Conversely, if the amount is too low, the treatment could be ineffective, with either of the outcome perhaps leading to organ rejection in time.

Yesterday, I needed to have these labs done to review the number of white blood cells in my bloodstream. Even a year out from the transplant, changes may still be required to my medications.

This type of bloodletting is far from being a big deal. It's merely part of the routine process of the life of a transplant patient. I expect these labs to be required for the rest of my life, with medications being added, removed, and adjusted throughout.

Having needles being plunged into my skinny arms, searching for that vein, which will inevitably roll once the skin is pierced, is certainly no fun. But it is surely better than the alternative.

#12 – September 25, 2018

Thirteen months ago this morning, I received the call that a donor had become available to provide me with fresh lungs and a liver.

This donor gave me the greatest gift of all - a future with a longer and better quality of life. I could not be more grateful for that precious gift. At the same time, I greatly mourn the donor family's loss of their loved one, as they just ended their first summer without their daughter/sister/wife/mother.

That family will forever be minus one.

Please consider becoming an organ donor. As of 12:38 pm EST today, there are 74,829 individuals who are active waiting list candidates. One person is added to the national transplant waiting list every ten minutes, and twenty-two people die every day while awaiting a transplant.

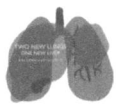

One donor can save eight lives and affect the lives of countless others. Every life saved creates a story for that person rescued. Take the opportunity to create eight stories.

It costs nothing to save a life. Live on through others and become a lifelong hero to many.

To register your decision to save and heal lives, visit RegisterMe. org. To learn more about organ, eye, tissue and living donation, visit DonateLife.net.

#13 – September 29, 2018

I was having dinner with a friend of mine and her boyfriend a few weeks back. She is a high school classmate, and we were just catching up. On her life and mine.

During our conversation, we talked about my life after the transplant, and how I've been able to travel like never before. I told my friend about how I have been taking road trips, have been flying here and there at a moment's notice. After speaking about these great experiences, my friend asked me what was next on my bucket list. And that made me pause.

I really couldn't answer her too well, and for a couple of reasons. I have always thought that a bucket list is something you want to do before you die. And I honestly never thought I was going to die. Cystic Fibrosis wasn't going to take me. Not a chance. So, I've never had a bucket list. I never saw a point in it.

But after some thought and quite a bit later, I began to think about all I can do now with these new lungs. And that, in itself, I now realize may have been my bucket list wish. My ultimate bucket list wish. To be able to travel, by air or by car, at the spur of the moment, without having to think about my meds – what I need to take with me, how much I need to take with me, calculating it all out, how will I store it in the hotel where I will be staying. Not to mention making sure I don't pack too much to ensure that I can still carry all my luggage, which include the vest and neb machines.

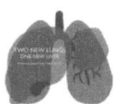

I am now living that new life. The reservations for the last two trips via flight were spur of the moment decisions. The first trip was a plan to fly back home to Hawaii, for which reservations were made five hours before the plane took off, and for the second trip, I booked a ticket the afternoon before departure the next morning. The last road trip I undertook lasted for 20 hours, driving nearly non-stop, and I decided to engage in that adventure 12 hours before I left.

So, while obtaining new lungs may not have been on my bucket list, per se, having a new life, a second life, one of freedom from the most burdensome effects of Cystic Fibrosis, may, in fact, subconsciously have been a bucket list wish. I never imagined, though, it could actually ever become a reality.

But thanks to my donor, I have now achieved that. My ultimate bucket list wish.

#14 – October 2, 2018

The other week, I had dinner with my doctor back home. It's always good to see him in a casual setting, now that the transplant has taken care of the pulmonary aspects of Cystic Fibrosis for me. Before, conversations focused on my declining, or at best stable, but still unacceptable, lung functions. And whether I want to go into the hospital for IVs or do them at home. These days, my meetings with him are merely times to sit, chat and eat.

During our meal, my doctor's cell phone rang. Turns out it was a call from a parent of one of his patients. It seemed that child of the person on the line was the typical patient that my doctor treats. Based on the words of my doctor, it seemed that the child, whether she has CF or not, was apparently feeling sick. What made the call meaningful for me were the words my doctor was using on this call to his patient.

"Does she feel like she's getting worse?" "Does she feel like she wants to start IVs, or does she want to wait?" "Okay. Go to the lab in the morning and have her provide a sputum sample, then I'll call you to see when she can come in." Those were the same words he used

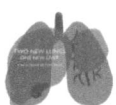

when talking to me over the years, as I was on the path to the eventual 17% lung function I had earned by the time I left my home in July 2017 prior to the transplant.

Listening to those same words as when they were said to me, time and time again, in my doctor's slow, calm and easy tone brought me back. His calming style of speech was always somewhat reassuring, both because he never gave the impression, regardless of how bad my health was at the time, that I was in dire need of IV treatments, and because I knew the routine of the steps he was describing. At my age of 44 at the time, I was aware of the procedures. The good and bad of the IVs, of being in the hospital for a two to three-week duration.

At the same time, there was always a touch of anxiety involved with that news. Knowing that by going into the hospital, I would be again missing work for an undetermined period of time, knowing the negative side effects of the IVs I would be dosed with for at least a fortnight, wondering how much pulmonary function I had lost since my last IV treatment not too long ago.

Although I would quickly get over those musings, as I had become a veteran of those battles, it is still not a place I wanted my mind to be.

This time, now being on the passive side of the words of my doctor, and knowing that I would likely never be hearing that type of guidance from my doctor again, was surreal. I could feel the cloud the parent at the other end of the conversation was under at the moment, because I remembered when those words were directed toward me.

But all the same, I felt relief. The relief one feels as a patient who 13 months ago received two new lungs and liver. The relief that it is entirely possible that I may never have to hear those words from my doctor ever again.

The feeling that I was beginning a new life. A new freedom. The feeling of gratitude toward my beautiful, generous donor. The one who made my second life, my new life, a true reality.

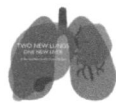

#15 – October 5, 2018

It was a few weeks back when I received a Facebook memory. A year ago, I posted a comment a nurse made when I was in rehab, recovering from the transplant I had a month earlier. When one of the floor nurses entered my room, she told me, "You smell like medication." That was about right.

Given that I was a month from the transplant, although I had been weaned from most of the meds I had been taking, I still had a good amount flowing into me. The way I looked at the smell the nurse experienced, it was not necessarily medication she noticed.

It was the smell of healing. It was the smell of the generosity of my donor who allowed me to use her lungs and liver. It was the smell of 45 years of daily treatments and increasing IV dosages due to Cystic Fibrosis fading away. It was the smell of dreams forming, dreams of doing things I could never have thought of experiencing with my original lungs due to my expected brief life that all CF patients endure.

The smell of my undertaking last minute, spur of the moment road trips and plane rides. The smell of endeavoring to achieve a private pilot's license. The smell of planning to age into retirement.

There was, indeed, a smell of something in my room that day. And it was a smell of medication, for certain. But it really was a smell of something deeper. Something more pervasive. It was the smell of a new beginning for me, the smell of a new life.

Further, just as important, and perhaps even deeper, it was the smell of enduring thanks and gratitude for the priceless gift my donor provided me. The smell of the unspoken lifetime bond she and I will always keep.

#16 – October 8, 2018

As unspeakably thankful as I am for the organs I received from my donor that enabled me to have a second chance at life, to allow me the opportunity to live a full and more robust life, I always keep in mind the family of my donor.

During those times when I think about who my donor was, what she did for a living, how old she was, what hobbies she used to enjoy, my mind inevitably gravitates to her family. In that square, I think about how they felt at the time when the doctors must have gingerly broken the news that their daughter, wife, mother was not going to make it. That her brain was no longer functioning. And permission was asked of the family whether her organs may be donated to someone in need.

I then attempt to juxtapose the family's feelings with mine at the time. When I had thoughts that tinged of hope. When I thought this transplant might actually work. That these lungs, that liver, could possibly change my life.

During a night in late August 2017, the life of a beautiful, caring, and giving lady ceased to be, and my second life was about to begin. As time passed, my body gradually accepted her life and her body into mine. I healed and became stronger.

In subsequent days, as I counted the hours and weeks of the commencement of my new life, her family experienced the first in a series of mornings and nights without this beautiful woman that will continue for an unending period.

From time to time, I submit the unanswerable question to myself: Is there a degree of measurement to determine whether the peak of my happiness for the opportunity to hope and chase dreams I never could before is higher than the depths of the trough of sadness, despair and grief that my donor's family feels now and will forever?

Unanswerable, indeed.

#17 – October 11, 2018

It was a couple of days ago that I was talking to a friend who also has Cystic Fibrosis. It turns out that she is in the middle of a typical exacerbation, which causes breathing difficulties, persistent coughing, and in some instances, blood is included with that cough. After having lived with CF for over forty years, I empathize with her and can absolutely re-

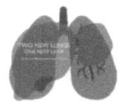

late to her situation. We were discussing the uncomfortable and, some would even say, nasty side effects of the medication named Zyvox.

I recognize how fortunate and blessed I am that since my transplant a bit over a year ago, at this time I no longer endure any treatments related to CF. More importantly, since the transplanted lungs do not contain the CF genes, I thankfully have no cause to develop the chronic lung infections I typically learned to expect and dealt with throughout my life, as do all individuals with Cystic Fibrosis.

At the same time, I wholly understand that these healthy lungs may not always remain this way. There is the constant threat of organ rejection, which could detrimentally affect my lungs and/or liver at any time. I am constantly aware of this. As a result, I also thank my lucky stars each and every day for my good health, knowing it could all change in a day. Or in a minute.

It is for that reason I take each day, to coin a phrase, one day at a time. Not a 24-hour period passes that I don't give thanks to my donor for the golden gifts she gave me.

At the end of the conversation I was having with my friend when we were commiserating over her current Zyvox treatments, I told her how I remembered the unpleasantries of that med, and how I used to hate taking it. The segment of that conversation ended with her responding with, "Isn't is amazing that you get to talk about it in past tense?"

It undoubtedly is.

#18 – October 14, 2018

I was talking to a friend the other day, and it turns out that we got onto the topic of organ donation. The conversation brought to light an aspect of organ donation I had previously never thought of.

On this side of an organ donation story, on the side of an organ recipient, of course I advocate for someone becoming an organ donor. To check the box. At the same time, I have always been aware that when that inevitable day arrives, and the donor's family is faced with the decision of granting their loved one's wish, it is a soul wrenching moment.

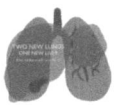

Before having this conversation with my friend, it never dawned on me what all the emotions might be when agreeing to transfer your loved one's organs to another. To grant their wish. Apart from what I have always considered to be the primary painful dilemma of providing the approval to end the life of your mother/father/wife/husband/sister/brother/daughter/son so that a stranger can take possession of his or her organs, and begin a second life, I had never recognized that there also might be an ethical dilemma regarding the transplant process – who will be organs be going to? Will they be transferred to that person for the right reasons? Will they be transferred to the right person, in general?

Deciding to donate our own organs, or the organs of someone we love, is a such a personal decision. In my view, there is no right or wrong. I will, of course, advocate each and every time for organ donation. For that cause. To give someone who is on the edge of their life a second chance. To give them a new beginning. At the same time, I understand and respect the views of those who cannot commit to organ donation for any number of reasons. Whether they be religious, cultural, or just strictly personal reasons.

Although this posting may sound like a lengthy random thought, I write this because the conversation I had made me appreciate even more the decision my donor's family made on that night. The night when her life was on the verge of entering the next phase, away from this world. When likely a complete stranger at the hospital asked her family on that night whether they could preserve and extend her life by giving it to someone else.

I am forever grateful that my donor's family said Yes. And that Yes gave me that second chance. That second life. The one that will always have me thanking her, and just as importantly, thanking her family for allowing my donor, this lady, to fulfill her wishes of giving back in the ultimate manner. In the ultimate way.

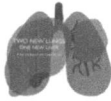

#19 – October 17, 2018

I went to a concert the other night, and it was an experience for more than just taking in a good performance. It was more because of the milestone in my health timeline that it allowed me to recognize and celebrate.

My trip to the concert venue began with a Lyft ride to the arena where the showing was being held. During the conversation with the driver, I told him which artist I was going to see, to which he responded, in a mildly surprised tone, "I wouldn't expect that *you* would be going there." He stated that expression twice, further enhancing his disbelief. I got to wondering what was so unbelievable about me attending that specific performance. Is it that I look old? Certainly not, because I am not. In addition to having Cystic Fibrosis, I also have Multiple Sclerosis. So, I walk with a cane. Was his belief based on the fact that I was going to the concert of a pop artist because I was handicapped? Certainly not, because I am certainly not that. Certainly not.

Moving beyond that situation, once I made it to the concert arena, I located my seats which were in the nosebleed section of the venue, some ten rows down from the very top. In the past, and with my old lungs, I would have dismissed outright the thought of going to that concert, strictly due to my seating location. Climbing those stairs would not have been an option. My damaged lungs would not have permitted that. Traversing the crowds and stepping up about twenty rows of stairs would have felt tantamount to climbing Mt. Everest with no oxygen pack. And with no Sherpa to assist.

The ultimate gratification for me was when I had reached my seat, on the aisle just off the stairs. I turned to sit, and in my field of view was a man who had been following me up the stairs, who must have been 10 flights back. He was apparently behind me as I ascended the stairs, as I grasped the railing with my left hand, carrying my cane with the right. He stood there looking at me with his mouth slightly opened, and with a look of astonishment. After a couple of seconds, he continued to climb past me, en route to his seat.

I, of course, was not able to talk to him. But if I had the chance, I would have told him the story about my donor. About how she checked

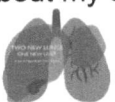

the box. About how when one night in late August of 2017, she encountered a terrible situation and lost her life. About how I received a call early on the morning of August 25th that told me they found a match. About how the voice on the other end of the call told me to get to the hospital immediately to receive my brand-new lungs and liver. My gift.

About how when her life ended, she extended mine. About how beautiful, generous, and caring that woman was.

And I would have asked him if he checked the box. Checked the box to become an organ donor, allowing a second chance to a stranger whose life is on the edge. If he had yet done that. If so, I would have thanked him.

And if he had not yet checked the box, I'd have ask him why not.

#20 – October 20, 2018

*M*y routines are now different.

For the first 44 years of my life, I endured and followed a certain schedule, as do all with Cystic Fibrosis. And followed it regularly. Upon waking, I would brush my teeth and shower. The next task was not breakfast, because that would have interrupted the flow. Treatments were my priority.

Treatments involved inhaling a series of nebulized medication while being hooked up to a machine that would shake and vibrate my torso. The machine called "The Vest" is well known to all Cystic Fibrosis patients. This process required that I wake at 4:00 each workday morning in order to successfully complete the treatments prior to heading to work. When I finished work, the first thing I did when I walked in the door was to repeat that same routine.

I'm detailing my past because today is one of those days when it struck me how different things are now with my new, non-CF lungs. For my entire life, I had to follow those treatments. Twice a day. Every day. Tired or not, they had to be done. Each session would take about an hour or so. Skipping those treatments too often, as I did far too often, would result in hospitalizations. Or home IVs.

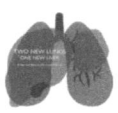

The damage which resulted from those missed treatments was what, in part, caused my lungs to function at only 17%. Missing those treatments caused me to be placed onto the lung transplant list in 2017. Missing those treatments caused my life to intersect with the wonderful lady who gave me her lungs.

I started this post saying that my routines are now different. As I now wake up each morning, I test my lung capacity with a small device termed a "spiro". I exhale forcefully into the spiro to make sure my lung capacity is not dipping to a level of concern. That's my new routine.

Every day for 44 years. This was my routine before with my old lungs. A one-hour treatment each morning. A one-hour treatment each night.

My treatment now with the new lungs gifted to me by my angel donor?

A five to ten-second breath into a device each morning. A thought and prayer to my donor for giving me these new lungs and liver each night.

#21 – October 23, 2018

Welcome to enhanced traveling, I tell myself.

Prior to my transplant nearly 14 months ago, and especially soon before the surgery, traveling was becoming a burden. One factor was my need to carry an oxygen concentrator with me on flights. For a time, I thought that was a foolish requirement. And unnecessary at that. Needing oxygen on a plane. That was dumb, I thought. Why?

My lung functions were at about 20% at best at the time, but I surmised that I'd be fine breathing oxygen on the plane just as all others could. Just like anyone else.

On one trip, I was midway through a flight and decided to check my oxygen level. Just for kicks. I found that my oxygen saturation was at 62%.

From then on, I brought with me not only the oxygen concentrator on every flight, but also enough batteries to last 150% of the flying time.

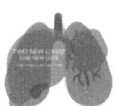

Since I lived in Hawaii at the time, a typical five or six-hour flight to the west coast meant that I had to take with me on my carry-on three three-hour batteries, which weighed two pounds each. If I wanted to travel beyond the west coast, I would need four batteries, weighting a total of eight pounds.

All in, considering the six to eight pounds of batteries in my backpack carry-on, I also had to stuff into that bag my nebulizer machine for the breathing treatments, aerosol meds and pills, a laptop and its power cord, and any other items I had to take with me that were too important to risk being lost in a misrouted suitcase.

Thinking back, and taking into account that I needed a cane at the time, although I was too stubborn to use one. Plus, I was too proud to use the wheelchair service to take me from ticket agent, through TSA, and to the gate.

So, there I was on each trip, focusing on walking so I didn't trip or topple over, carrying a backpack that weighed easily at least 15 pounds, and with my lungs functioning at between 17% and 20%. All of this without using my oxygen, because I refused to allow people to see me in a public place with a cannula under my nose. Lest they think I might be handicapped. Or that there was something wrong with me.

Or worse yet – Not Normal. Because I was absolutely normal. Absolutely.

I now bring myself back to a few days ago, when I returned home to Hawaii. Taking the long walk on the way from the ticket gate to the boarding area, which I used to truly and clearly dread in a way that would be unimaginable if I attempted to describe it.

Now with two new lungs, gifted to me by my beautiful donor, I walked slowly with my cane, enjoying the light Hawaiian breeze, taking in the sights of the majestic 767s and 757s parked nearby at the gates. I was finally able to take pleasure in that walk.

I then allowed myself a moment to think back to the times with my old lungs. How I struggled to make that beautiful walk, in which I could find absolutely no beauty or joy.

In that instance, I formed a "thank you" in my thoughts. It was to my donor.

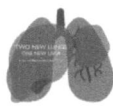

And I wondered if she was watching me walk. And I wondered if she was smiling. And I wondered if she responded to my thoughts with a gentle "you are welcome".

Perhaps she did. Perhaps.

#22 – October 25, 2018

Fourteen months ago this morning, I received the call that a donor had become available to provide me with fresh lungs and a liver.

This donor gave me the greatest gift of all - a future with a longer and better quality of life. I could not be more grateful for that precious gift. At the same time, I greatly mourn the donor family's loss of their loved one. If my wonderful donor had small children, this is the second time their mother will not be there to dress them for Halloween. She will again be unable to hold their hands as they walk their neighborhood and share their joy on what is supposed to be an evening of enjoyment, fun, and memories.

That family will forever be minus one.

Please consider becoming an organ donor. As of 11:57 am EST today, there are 75,078 individuals who are active waiting list candidates. One person is added to the national transplant waiting list every ten minutes, and twenty-two people die every day while awaiting a transplant.

One donor can save eight lives and affect the lives of countless others. Every life saved creates a story for that person rescued. Take the opportunity to create eight stories.

It costs nothing to save a life. Live on through others and become a lifelong hero to many.

#23 – October 31, 2018

Most thoughts about someone receiving an organ transplant involve the person being grateful for the opportunity to live a longer life.

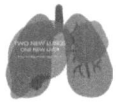

So that they can be healthier and feel well enough to live a fuller life. That is indeed a benefit, truly. However, I witnessed another benefit to having a second chance at life, the opportunity at a longer, fuller life, when my mother passed away last week.

As any family with a person diagnosed with Cystic Fibrosis years ago can attest, it was generally accepted that the child will pass away prior to the parents. Given that I was born in the early 1970s, when having CF meant a sure death sentence, it was always my mindset that I would go first. Although I never broached the topic with my parents, I can easily assume they expected the same.

However, that expectation seemed to possibly change when I received a fresh set of lungs and a liver from a beautiful donor in August 2017. It was nowhere near the top of my mind that since I no longer have CF in my lungs, and I now have a fresh start, that I may now outlive my parents. Not near the top of my mind, but it was certainly on the fringe.

As it happened, that exact reality struck me two weeks ago when I received a text from my brother, informing me of my mother's failing health. He encouraged me to fly home, so we could be with her in case anything went astray with her situation. It was six days later that her situation did go astray, and she passed from us.

Among my thoughts in the hours and days subsequent to my mother's departure was that regardless of the pain and loss I felt from losing my mom, I realized two things

As much as I was suffering at the time, I realized that the trauma of a parent losing her child would have been far greater than what I was enduring. That a parent burying a child would likely be the toughest duty any parent would ever have to realize. That it is likely that the pain of never being able to witness a child grow, succeed, and engage in all the wonders life has to offer would not only be grossly unfair, but would be wholly devastating.

Further, I was able to realize the painful, dark, and yet somehow beautiful experience I had with my brother, as we sat by our mother's side during her last hours, during her last minutes, during her last seconds. Our presence enabled her last moments on this earth to be with

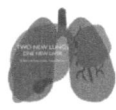

her two sons. Accordingly, my brother's face and mine were the last sights she witnessed as she left this world.

That last moment on a Wednesday morning at 3:36 was the beauty among the pain and the darkness.

That beauty was made possible exclusively by my donor, who allowed me her organs, so I could be with my mother when it mattered the most.

Before she passed, I asked my mom to say "hello" to my donor, should she see her on the other side. If my mom does see her, I wonder if she, too, will thank my donor for allowing her that same beauty.

#24 – November 3, 2018

When I think about my donor who gave me a second chance at life, I always try to take a chance to pause, think about, and thank her family and those of other angel donors. Without the family's desire to grant the donor's wish to pass their life onto the next, the donations could not be realized, and the gifts could not be granted.

The other day, I had a conversation with a lady whose mother was a donor, and the talk further brought the above point home to me.

It was a call to my insurance company, and I was speaking with a woman about my current condition post-transplant. We began a conversation about my transplant, about my situation in the years leading up to the transplant, the time of the transplant, and of my life since. I shared with her how much my world has changed for the better since I received the gifts from my donor.

During our discussion, this lady confided in me that her mother passed away unexpectedly years ago, and that she was asked whether she would be willing to donate her mother's organs. She told me about how she struggled over the decision, as her mother had not indicated a desire either way. In the end, this lady chose to share her mother's organs.

She told me that the organ donor network she worked with provided her a letter detailing to whom her mother's organs were given. This

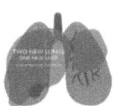

lady shared with me her recollection of the correspondence which stated her mother's eyes were donated to a recipient in France, as there was no candidate available in her region at that time.

Toward the end of our talk, this lady thanked me for telling my story. She confided in me that she had spent the past 15 years feeling torn inside, always debating whether she had made the right decision in allowing her mother to be taken from her in that way.

But she listened to my journey, about how I went from 17% lung function and dependent upon oxygen for many of my days, to now realizing 99% to 100% oxygen saturation. About how I had not been able to shop for groceries back then because of insufficient oxygen intake. About how I had been burdened with an oxygen concentrator when traveling, and to some extent not being able to travel as I pleased, to now flying on a commercial plane on a whim without limitations, and even taking a lesson to pilot a plane myself. About how I went from a Cystic Fibrosis patient with a life expectancy of 10 years in the early 1970s, to now anticipating a nearly normal life expectancy.

This lady told me that after our conversation, given what she learned, she was finally at peace with her decision to allow a second chance to needy strangers through her mother.

While our talk seemed to finally allow her mind to rest, our talk left me feeling thankful as well. Thankful to this lady for allowing her mom to save others, and thankful to my donor for giving me a chance not only to live, but also a chance to share my story about my wonderful and beautiful donor, thereby easing the unrest of another beautiful and giving soul.

#25 – November 6, 2018

Fall is here. Winter is approaching. This leads to the time when the weather becomes nippy here in Texas. The other morning, I had been up for a bit, but had not yet turned on the heat in my room.

At one point, I felt that my hands were cold, so I looked at them and saw that my fingernails had a purple tinge. It was, of course, an easy fix

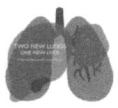

to warm my hands. To get the fingernails back to their normal color of pink.

However, that moment took me back. It took me back to a time beginning over and a half ago when my fingernails were purple, because I did not have enough oxygen in my bloodstream. Because my lungs were failing.

I was told by my doctor more than once in 2017 that my lips and fingernails were purple during what were becoming more frequent visits to him. I would always deny that anything about me had a purple tinge to it, even when it was clearly occurring.

To admit that fact would be to admit that there was something wrong. To admit that my lungs truly may be functioning at 17%. To admit the machine that displayed the reading really was working. To admit that results were low not just because I was tired. To admit that I really did need to use oxygen.

I couldn't admit any of that, because there was nothing wrong with me. I was convinced I was going to live longer than Moses. Not a metaphor. I was convinced that I was going to live forever.

If not for my beautiful donor, my lips and fingernails would have become increasingly purple. And it would have gotten to the point where I would have had to admit everything I never wanted to admit. That I truly was sick.

That my lungs were truly being destroyed minute by minute, hour by hour, day by day.

As a result of my generous and wonderful donor, my lips and fingernails are pink again. Also because of her, they are remaining that way.

#26 – November 9, 2018

It was a few days back when I was awaiting a prescription at CVS. As I allowed my eyes to wander upon the offerings in the shelves near the checkout counter, they focused on the plethora of probiotics at the highest level of the display. My mind fixated on those. To me, in the

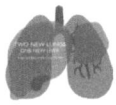

months leading up to the transplant, I looked at probiotics as one of my vital and essential lifelines.

Resulting from the potent antibiotics I was taking in an increasingly desperate effort to maintain pulmonary health, and to keep my lung function from falling below the 17% where it was at the time, it was a constant struggle to keep my digestive system under control. I would always search for the brand of probiotics that would serve me best, always attempting to identify exactly which cultures would battle those dysfunctions successfully.

Several text and messaging discussions with my brother to probe his knowledge of the subject. Carefully and repeatedly studying the note my doctor gave me that listed the most helpful bacteria for my case. Having to learn that the probiotic which contained 20 billion live cultures is not necessarily better than the one that contained 11 billion.

The unfortunate purchases of the incorrect type taught me this regrettable lesson too many times.

Although the endless quest and hunt I undertook to find the correct brand and strength may seem to be a trivial matter to some, when it dictated what I was able to do day by day, discouraging me from leaving my apartment to take in some enjoyment, steering my mind away during work too many times since I always had to be mindful of my gut, lest the unfortunate occur unexpectedly, it was indeed most paramount.

The wrong choice was certain to provide much stress, worry and, well, you can imagine what else, until I decided to return to the pharmacy and experiment with a different strain.

It is something as simple as viewing a selection of digestive aides that makes me think about my wonderful donor. She not only gave me lungs that enabled me to breathe, thereby extending my life. She provided me with a better quality of life as well.

New lungs meant no antibiotics. It meant no probiotics. It meant no frantic bathroom emergencies.

It meant a new life.

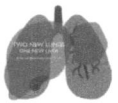

#27 – November 12, 2018

I was talking to someone the other day. We quickly came upon the topic of my health.

This person knew that I have Cystic Fibrosis. Therefore, she was knowledgeable about the inherently dire situation those of us with CF are faced with from day one. She knew about the short-predicted life span of those who have CF, particularly those who were born decades ago. I shared with her that my parents were told by doctors that I would not live past the age of 10.

At the same time, she knew about my transplants. She knew how well I have been doing because of the organs I received from my donor. She knew how lucky I feel, and how I know how fortunate I am.

As the conversation progressed, due to my new, gifted organs, she implied that it is more likely now that I will live close to a normal life span. I agreed, but I told her that in the past, I surely did not see any path to that type of outcome.

In younger years, I had focused on the anticipated expected life spans. I thought CF would initiate my early demise at the age of 23. Surpassing that age, I thought my next year of expiration would be 29. When I outlived that mark, I was absolutely convinced that I would be gone by the age of 31. That was 15 years ago.

I told her that I had been preparing to die for 25 years.

About a week later, I was messaging a friend who also has CF. We got to chatting about how far things have advanced with CF treatments. About how these improvements had led to the reality of longer life spans for those of us within our community.

Reflecting the grim statistics allocated to CF patients in the past, my friend said she had been preparing to die all these years.

This made me think about my donor and all the beautiful donors who enable life extensions to CF patients through their unselfish gifts. Gifts to the multitude of us who have been planning to die early throughout our lives, before organ transplants become a legitimate reality.

Although there was no way for the donors to know that their organs were going to be granted to someone with CF at the end of their journey, they had to know their organs would serve as a lifesaving opportunity for someone in need. They couldn't have helped but know what they had was of value. To know it was something so worthy that it would provide some unknown stranger a second chance.

And I am forever grateful they knew.

#28 – November 15, 2018

I tend to be a morning person.

I enjoy leaving my place at an early hour, whether it be to travel to work or to exercise at the gym. I appreciate being on the road when no or few other cars are venturing out. At the same time, in the darkness of the pre-dawn, at the most peaceful point of the day, my mind wanders toward my donor.

Was she doing the same as I often do, savoring a quiet drive in the early morning on an empty road, when her silence was shattered by a horrible collision? When both her morning tranquility and her life were immediately halted in a moment? In a split second. In an instant.

I do not yet know of the circumstances behind the passing of my donor. It's possible that I may never know.

I may never know what was happening in the wee hours of August 25th. At the time when I was sleeping in a motel room, awaiting a donor to become available. When I was talking to my dad about an hour before I received the call from the hospital informing me that there was indeed a donor available.

When I reassured my dad that it was okay that I hadn't yet received a call. Because every day I waited for that donor to be found meant another day of life for that unknown person who was predestined to become my donor.

I may never know the action which preceded and initiated the call I received at approximately 7:20 am, advising me to make my way to the hospital ASAP.

My donor certainly could not have known the day of her passing, and what the circumstances of that situation would be. But I truly owe

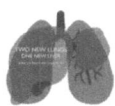

her my life and will always be grateful that she made the decision to extend her life through a stranger whom she would never meet.

It is for that reason my early morning drives will always be special to me. It allows me the time to feel as close as I can be to this wonderful woman who unknowingly saved my life.

#29 – November 18, 2018

It was something I had been hoping to receive. The other night, I was fortunate to receive a letter from my donor's family. Specifically, from my donor's mother.

When I saw the envelope on the counter, I knew immediately what it contained.

I sat on the side of my bed, holding the envelope. I needed to convince myself to open it. The content was what I had been waiting for, hoping for, since the beginning days of my new lungs, my new liver, my new life. At the same time, I was hesitant.

I knew once I read the letter, a new chapter would begin in my life. I would finally learn of the tale of a beautiful person who gave me a new life, a second chance, a brand-new future. Someone I would have never known, but now know and have a bond with through fate.

Having opened the envelope, I sat with the letter in one hand, the other hand covering my face which must have expressed a mixed view of hope, excitement, and apprehension. For a brief few moments. Then I started reading.

The words written on those pages reflected the life of a beautiful young lady who I had been hoping to learn about for nearly 15 months. The name of my angel is Joni Marie.

Joni Marie's mother told me of the two young and incredible children my donor tragically left behind. I began to think about their first Thanksgiving last year without their mother. Their first Christmas last year without their mother. The start of their first year without their mother. I began to think about the emotional pain that must have caused

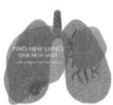

them. The grief I can't even imagine of the little ones being without the most important person in their lives.

It is my sincere hope that Joni Marie's children will one day know what a hero she is to me. The hero that I thought could never be found. My doctors would only accept for me a person who had nothing but the best liver and the best lungs. I did not at all think it was possible that such a person could be located.

Just a couple of days after the surgery, I was told that my donor's liver was the cleanest liver one of the surgeons had ever seen, and that both the lung and liver surgeons said, "whoever gets this donor will be very lucky."

How did it become that I was the lucky one to be graced with the great luck, fortune and blessing to have my path cross with that of Joni Marie?

There is no way I will ever know. But what I do know is that I would like to thank the children of Joni Marie for having such a caring, generous and gracious mother who allowed me to live another day. For her children to know the gifts she provided me, to live another year, to live another decade and beyond, are appreciated more than can be recognized.

And that their mother lives on. Through me and through all the several who are touched by her benevolent action.

And that the scope of their mother's actions is immeasurable. That it is inspiring. That it is the actions of an angel. A true angel.

#30 – November 25, 2018

Fifteen months ago this morning, I received the call that a donor had become available to provide me with fresh lungs and a liver.

My donor, Joni Marie, gave me the greatest gift of all - a future of a longer and better quality of life. I could not be more grateful for that precious gift. At the same time, I greatly mourn the donor family's loss of their loved one. Joni Marie had two small children. This past Thanksgiving was the second time their mother was not with them at the dinner

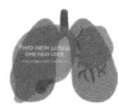

table, and the second time Joni Marie's parents and brother could not share with her what they have been thankful for this past year.

That family will forever be minus one.

Please consider becoming an organ donor. As of 11:46 am EST to-day, there are 75,181 individuals who are active waiting list candidates. One person is added to the national transplant waiting list every ten minutes, and twenty-two people die every day while awaiting a transplant.

One donor can save eight lives, and affect the lives of countless others. Every life saved creates a story for that person rescued. Take the opportunity to create eight stories.

It costs nothing to save a life. Live on through others, and become a lifelong hero to many.

#31 – November 28, 2018

It was the drive that almost didn't happen.

As I embarked on what turned out to be a 2,306 mile drive to spend Thanksgiving with my brother, it ran through my mind that the adventure I was about to undertake was not supposed to happen a mere 15 months ago, when I was waiting for an organ donor.

I thought about my donor, Joni Marie, who just two years ago was enjoying the Thanksgiving holidays with her two young children, her brother, and her parents. When I was setting out for my journey on the Tuesday prior to the holiday, it was two years ago that Joni Marie was likely thinking about how the turkey was going to be prepared. About when she had to thaw the turkey on which she and her family were going to feast.

I wonder if she was going to use canned cranberry sauce, or did she have a special secret recipe that was a favorite of her little boy and girl. Was she shopping on that day two years earlier for the ingredients for a pie that her parents looked forward to every year? Or was her brother going to take care of those preparations?

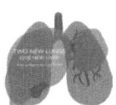

Driving between Dallas, TX and Scottsdale, AZ, playing lane-changing hopscotch with the other vehicles on the two and four-lane country highways that were being driven by those who were looking forward to Thanksgiving just as Joni Marie was a couple of years back, was another moment for me to ponder how lucky I am that my paths crossed with that of Joni Marie.

Two years ago, I did not think I needed a lung, let alone a liver, transplant. I was certain that I was sick but was sure I would be fine with routine hospitalizations and IV treatments every other month or so, using oxygen whenever I felt I absolutely had to.

Two years ago, Joni Marie did not think about the fact that I needed a lung, let alone a liver, transplant, either. She was certain that she would spend the next several decades with her family, watching her children grow, graduate from high school, then college. Witness her children begin their careers, find someone special, get engaged, get married. And at some point, enabling Joni Marie to be a grandmother. Baby-sitting her grandchildren as much as she could.

Two years ago, these were our separate situations.

Two years later, I am driving to my brother's place for a memorable Thanksgiving dinner.

Those same two years later, I am writing a blog thanking Joni Marie for checking the box, thereby saving my life. And thinking about the family she left behind on this past Thanksgiving holiday.

#32 – December 1, 2018

81%. What does that mean? Well, it kind of means a lot.

PFTs, or Pulmonary Function Tests, is the barometer, is the mile marker, for all Cystic Fibrosis patients. It's what you take at each doctor appointment. It's what you talk about with other CFers when you want to share your progress with this disease, whether it is positive or not. It's what contributes to the trend to chronicle whether you're improving. Or not.

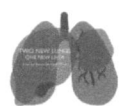

In my younger years, I remember my PFTs being in the 80s, then in the 70s. They were declining, but it wasn't any big deal to me. Not a big thing at all. This was in the 1980s, in the 1990s, in the early 2000s. I have Cystic Fibrosis. I knew what that meant, as did all others with CF at the time. CF is a disease that destroys the lungs. It eats away at the lung tissue bit by bit, year by year. As a result, our PFTs decline at a rate that is expected and understandable to us.

Similar to that of a cement truck rolling downhill on a moderate slope that has somehow gotten away from its driver. You know the truck will continue to rumble down that road, because there is simply not any force that can stop it. The pace of that truck will increase steadily until it encounters that barrier at the end of the path.

You will watch the truck speed downhill. You know what the end result will be. You lay spike strips onto the road to slow the decent. But you know the inevitable.

And as a CF patient, although it is not okay that the truck will be destroyed in the end, it is what you expect. You have seen this happen to others in the CF Community all your life. It was, frankly, reality to CFers in those times. In the 1980s, in the 1990s, in the early 2000s. And it was okay, because it had to be okay. It was life.

That was the circumstance with me, as well. I had laid down a numerous series of spike strips onto my road of life to slow the progress of CF over my decades of living, but I knew what the end would be. So, when my PFTs advanced into 25% lung function in the late 2000s, I was not surprised. It was the cement truck effect in full force.

It was unfortunate, certainly. But it was understandable. And expected. It was okay, because I still planned to continue to lay down spike strips until the useful life of that doomed cement truck came to its predetermined end. Whenever it would be. The truck's momentum would degenerate to PFTs of 20%, eventually to 17%. But it was okay. It was expected.

Then came August 2017, and my path crossed with that of my donor, Joni Marie. I was told that she could stop the acceleration of that runaway cement truck. I did not believe it. In my mind, although my truck would continue to roll to its eventual end, it was all right with me.

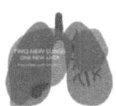

New lungs or not, I never expected the decline to cease. And that was okay. I had been expecting that outcome throughout my life.

I fast forward to my 15-month post-transplant appointment with my care team the other day. In keeping with tradition, I took my PFTs. The reading was 81%.

81%. It is an unspoken non-belief to me. I was at 17% in August of 2017. I needed oxygen at that point. Fifteen months later, I am at 81%.

I think any words to describe my feeling of a new life at 81% would be trivial. I just think about Joni Marie. I think about her lungs that are now a part of me. The lungs responsible for an 81%.

And I thank Joni Marie for her gift. And I always will. Rest in Peace, Joni Marie.

#33 – December 4, 2018

The anxiety of having to undergo an organ transplant does not begin at the time the person is listed for the transplant. Indeed, it begins well prior.

The other day, I saw a post from a friend on Facebook who was reflecting on her pending transplant status. She is on the brink of being placed onto the list. That brink in her situation, as it is with many pre-transplantees, is not desirable.

My friend has Cystic Fibrosis and has been dealing with the condition and its extremes all her life. The frequent hospitalizations. The IV treatments. The lung damage. The loss of lung function.

Several years ago, her doctors considered placing her onto the organ transplant list. For various reasons, she was not included on that unenviable list at the time. However, circumstances are such that her health has continued to decline, and she is now once more on the verge of becoming a candidate for placement.

As it stands, the current dilemma is that although she is unwell, in fact, she is very sick, my friend's lung function may have improved to an extent where she is not a candidate for a transplant at this time. That reality brings about many dismal factors.

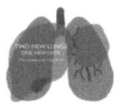

If one is sick enough so that the conversation of being placed on the list is inaugurated, it means that the body is struggling to function. This brings about constant fatigue. It brings about constant coughing fits. Coughing up blood.

It brings about a feeling that you are drowning in your own mucus. It brings about body pains, body aches. It brings about the necessity of hospital admissions, together with several intrusive treatments and therapies each day that intrude upon the normalcy of life.

At this point, a lung transplant, as severe and as traumatic as it is, regardless of the uncertainty and anxiety it would cause, would offer a welcome respite from the trials and pain that has been a part of the patient's world for many several years.

I experienced the above plights of discomfort during the six months prior to my transplant last year. So much, that I think of not only my friend who is in the forlorn situation of needing to be just a little sicker than she already is in order to be invited the opportunity to become an organ transplantee, but I think of my donor, Joni Marie, for checking the box, for the unselfish deed of offering herself to someone at the end of her time. For allowing me the opportunity to breathe without the feeling of drowning from inside. For giving me that second chance.

And I think of my friend who is lingering on the edge of a lung transplant. Awaiting the time when her second chance can commence. Awaiting the time when she no longer feels as if she is drowning from the inside.

Awaiting her rescue. Awaiting her angel. Awaiting her Joni Marie.

#34 – December 7, 2018

I'm currently in Las Vegas to celebrate my brother's 50th Birthday. In traveling here, I took an airplane. Being on a plane now always makes me think of the simplest, yet the most obvious, element. Oxygen. And how breathing it in is not always automatic.

As is the case with a good number of us with Cystic Fibrosis, for several months prior to my transplant, I was encouraged to use oxy-

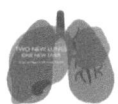

gen. During the last few months prior to receiving the gift of lungs from my angel donor Joni Marie, without the use of external oxygen, my oxygen was reading at about 87% to 90% when at rest. Certainly, the level of O2 declined when I would move.

Eventually, it became so I could no longer shop for groceries. I was too stubborn to use an oxygen concentrator outside my apartment, because anyone noticing me with it would recognize that there was something wrong. And that was simply not allowed to be the case.

Because of my inadequate oxygen level, it was too taxing for me to push the cart at Costco, heavily laden with goods. Guiding it along the aisles was difficult enough, but the most challenging was traversing the parking lot over the uneven asphalt. That exhausted me more than I could have ever previously imagined.

Not to mention placing the groceries into my car, then carrying it up to my apartment once I got home. The vast majority of goods would remain in the car's trunk for days, sometimes even weeks, because I was only physically able to carry one item at a time.

Even retrieving my prescriptions was becoming too much. There was a slight incline in the parking lot leading to the CVS store. Hiking that path would literally take my breath away. I needed to utilize a shopping cart to ascend that minimal slope, because it was my guide for balance. Although I had usually one small package containing maybe two or three small bottles of meds, the usage of the cart was imperative in order to keep from tumbling, given I often became lightheaded from the activity of walking through a drug store.

Perhaps the most memorable event compounded from insufficient oxygen came about when I was on a dinner run after work one night. When the phone app I was using notified me that Popeye's on Dillingham Boulevard was directly to my left, across two lanes of oncoming traffic, I made an immediate left turn without thought. Absent my looking to see where I was turning.

As it happened, when I passed through the two lanes, I noticed there was not any sort of opening in the street to turn into. There was instead a sidewalk directly ahead of me. Seeing out of the corner of my eye the several headlights quickly bearing down upon me, com-

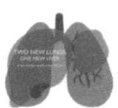

manding my inner Dukes of Hazard, I sped up and drove my Honda Civic over the sidewalk, scraping the undercarriage in the process, but thankfully avoiding the auto getting hung up on the curb, and entered the parking lot of the strip mall.

Recalling the situation with my doctor several days later, he surmised the oxygen insufficiency I had been experiencing that it was the lack of concentration, clear thinking and focus that caused that situation.

Bringing me back to the opening of this post, in my pre-transplant days, in order to fly, it was imperative that I had in tow an oxygen concentrator, accompanied by several heavy and burdensome batteries to ensure adequate oxygen flow throughout my flight.

When I boarded the aircraft on Thursday, I carried but a backpack.

It is safe to say that when Joni Marie, my angel donor, checked the box to allow her organs to be shared with someone at the end of her life, she had no idea what an invaluable asset, what a tremendous gift, her lungs could become to someone.

Joni Marie did not know I could no longer shop. She did not know how much of an inconvenience traveling had become for me.

She had no idea that I was nearly involved in what could have been a terrible auto accident due to my inability to think properly because of my low oxygen level.

Joni Marie didn't know what a gift she had to give. She didn't know someone needed her lungs. She didn't know I needed her lungs. But she checked the box anyway.

She didn't even know.

#35 – December 25, 2018

Sixteen months ago this morning, I received the call that a donor had become available to provide me with fresh lungs and a liver.

My donor, Joni Marie, gave me the greatest gift of all - a future with a longer and better quality of life. I could not be more grateful for that

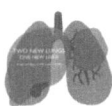

precious gift. At the same time, I greatly mourn the donor family's loss of their loved one.

Joni Marie has two small children, and today is the second time their mother is not with them on Christmas morning. Joni Marie is not there to watch them excitedly open their gifts. Joni Marie is not there to receive their thankful hugs. Joni Marie is not there to beam with joy, knowing how happy her little boy and girl are on this morning.

Today is the second time Joni Marie's parents and brother could not share with her what they have been thankful for this past year. They cannot share with Joni Marie their plans for the New Year.

Christmas will never be the same for them. Without their mother. Without their daughter and sister.

That family will forever be minus one.

Please consider becoming an organ donor. As of 9:57 am EST today, there are 75,134 individuals who are active waiting list candidates. One person is added to the national transplant waiting list every ten minutes, and twenty-two people die every day while awaiting a transplant.

One donor can save eight lives and affect the lives of countless others. Every life saved creates a story for that person rescued. Take the opportunity to create eight stories.

It costs nothing to save a life. Live on through others, and become a lifelong hero to many.

#36 – December 31, 2018

It was last week when I spent some time with an old friend of mine. She is the mother of a little girl who had Cystic Fibrosis and passed away far too early, nearly two weeks before her 19th birthday. Jenna left us five years ago, but it truly seems to me that it could not have been more than a year before.

Jenna's mother and I reminisced about the many years the three of us had as friends. We talked about Jenna's trials with CF. About her many bouts with this condition and its related complications from the

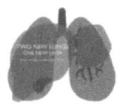

age of two years. Jenna's mom shared with me the frustrations experi-enced by her daughter, with the disease, and with certain things CF.

These frustrations are nothing new to anyone who has battled Cystic Fibrosis, but the nuances seemed especially fresh, somewhat painful, and absolutely regrettable to me. It was new to hear these agonizing stories from the parent of someone with CF. A parent who battled these obstacles, and fought to take down those barriers, for and with her child, only to lose her little girl just before she was to enter adulthood.

Our conversations that evening also brought back all sorts of mem-ories of my times before I was fortunate to have crossed paths with my Angel Donor, Joni Marie. Jenna's mother reminded me of when I used to post pictures of my IV medicine balls for the home infusions I had to undergo from time to time. It made me recall choosing to attend work while administering the IVs at my desk, in an effort to appear medically normal, instead of calling in sick to work because CF was trying to get the best of me.

I was reminded of the 25% lung function I held on to for about six years, before declining to 17% during my last year prior to the trans-plant. I was reminded of hesitating to use oxygen from the concentra-tor I had by my side at work, just in case. The one I would never, ever would use in public, even through bouts of feeling light-headed when walking, causing myself to trip and fall a time or two on the sidewalk, because I was concentrating more on breathing than I was on lifting my left foot.

Ultimately, all of this reminds me of the gift of life which my Angel Donor, Joni Marie, provided me when she passed one night on the last week of August 2017. It reminds me of the call I received from the hospital early the next morning, advising me to travel there ASAP. That they had found a donor. Someone to provide me with a second chance.

These memories and recollections of that time spent with Jenna's mother brought back two things in my mind.

One was the reminder of the awesome strength and courage Jenna displayed, and the examples she set as a young lady gracefully, fear-lessly and tirelessly battling CF at such an early age.

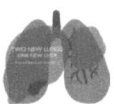

The other is of my Angel Donor, Joni Marie. The one who checked the box. The one who ensured I would be rescued from the future perils of CF with her decision to donate her organs once she no longer had a need for them.

The one who I think of each time I hear of those with CF who are battling to make it through their days. Each time I hear of those with CF whose battles with that disease have ended after having fought, but truly having never lost, the endless struggle.

It reminds me of my wish that each one of those Warriors will find their own Joni Marie one day soon.

And for those who passed from us well before their time, I truly wish they could have had their own Joni Marie, who would have saved them, too.

#37 – January 12, 2019

I had to change my mindset.

When I had my transplant almost a year and a half ago, I thought the many, many years of IV antibiotics were over for good. That the needles of the PICC line which had scarred the veins of one arm so badly that only the right could be used was a thing of the past. No more sticks. No more searching for veins. No more navigating around and over scar tissue to place the needle just so into a vessel leading into the heart.

Then I caught a cold.

I was on a road trip at the time, and I knew the perils a cold could cause the lungs of Joni Marie, my angel donor. With that in mind, as I drove through a snowstorm in New Mexico, I would find a reasonably sized shoulder along Highway 380, Highway 84, Highway 60. Along I-25. I would verify that no autos or 18-wheelers were approaching, swing open my door, and conduct various nasal rinses in hopes that the cold would not reach my lungs.

As time went on, it became clear through reduced spiro readings and an increased cough that the cold had indeed traveled to my lungs.

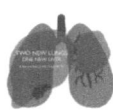

A visit to my doctor confirmed that I would be undergoing my first IV treatment post-transplant.

Admittedly, I was at first disappointed. I thought after the transplant that I would never again have to find ways to deal with the two or three med IV treatments. Having to start an IV, lie down to sleep after setting the alarm so I would awake in an hour and a half to disconnect the IV, only to wake up at 2:00 am to start another IV, soon followed by the 2:30 am alarm to disconnect. And so on.

But I had to change my mindset.

Although I now realize it's possible that I may need to be on IVs regularly should I catch a bad cold in the future, I have to choose to look at the bigger picture.

With my original lungs that had CF, for 44 years, I was subject to treatments at least twice a day, each day. I would cough continuously each day, even when I wasn't sick. Knowing that each hospitalization and IV treatment was bringing me closer to a situation which I refused to believe could happen but recognizing that it one day may.

Now that I have been blessed to cross paths with my angel donor, Joni Marie, I no longer have CF lungs. Once this cold leaves me, I will no longer cough. This is something that someone who has CF cannot even fathom. And even though I may have to be on IVs every so often going forward, I will not have to ponder if the next IV treatment and hospitalization could be leading to an early end.

As I soon travel back home to Hawaii to lay my mother's ashes to rest, coughing or not, on IVs or not, I am thankful that I am still here to take care of my mother. Thanks to Joni Marie and her lungs.

So, I have changed my mindset.

I realize that my job now is to take care of these beautiful lungs my angel donor, Joni Marie, left me. And if the IVs are allowing me to do that, I am happy for the opportunity.

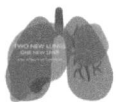

#38 – January 25, 2019

Seventeen months ago this morning, I received the call that a donor had become available to provide me with fresh lungs and a liver.

My donor, Joni Marie, gave me the greatest gift of all - a future with a longer and better quality of life. I could not be more grateful for that precious gift. At the same time, I greatly mourn her family's loss of their loved one.

This is the second time that Joni Marie's family is beginning their year without their daughter/mother/sister/wife. Her two small children will never again on midnight of December 31st look forward to celebrating another new year with their mom.

The New Year celebration will never be the same for them. Without their daughter and mother. Without their sister and wife.

That family will forever be minus one.

Please consider becoming an organ donor. As of 2:54 am EST today, there are 74,644 individuals who are active waiting list candidates. One person is added to the national transplant waiting list every ten minutes, and twenty people die every day while awaiting a transplant.

One donor can save eight lives and affect the lives of countless others. Every life saved creates a story for that person rescued. Take the opportunity to create eight stories.

It costs nothing to save a life. Live on through others, and become a lifelong hero to many.

In 2018, 36,527 organ transplants were performed from 17,555 donors. Become an organ donor, and become part of the story.

#39 – January 27, 2019

Flying back home from Hawaii last week to rest my mother's ashes, something came to mind.

Our mothers bring us into this world. It is they who look after our needs as we grow. From our first glop of baby formula to our first bowl of Fruit Loops. From our first pair of diapers to our first pair of corduroy pants we wore in second grade. From our first driving lesson to our first fender bender, when she stood by as we insisted to the responding officer that the other driver cut us off. When, in reality, that is not at all how it went down.

Staring out into the expansive Pacific, focusing on the clouds that dotted the ocean landscape, I realized that I owe my life to two women. Not only to my mother, but also to my angel donor, Joni Marie.

My mother brought me into the world as a fresh person. I was brand new, but with the catch that I had defective lungs. Growing up, my mother taught me how to take care of those lungs to get the most out of them. She made me exercise twice a day. She made me do treatments twice a day. She stressed that despite my having Cystic Fibrosis and MS, I could do and be anything I wanted.

At the middle of my fourth decade of life, she hoped I would get a lung transplant. That's where my angel donor came in.

In my mid-40s, despite how much my mother did to help me to keep my lungs healthy and fresh when I was young, and despite my efforts to do the same as an adult, CF took its toll. The damage became too much for the lungs to function at an optimal level. They declined to the point where a lung and liver transplant was needed.

That's where my angel donor, Joni Marie, came in.

As I looked over the expanse at 35,000 feet on my way to take care of my mom for the last time, I realized clearly for the first time that I had two women in my past who gave me life.

My mother gave me life at the beginning of mine.

Joni Marie gave me life when my lungs almost ceased to function. Joni Marie gave me life when mine was nearing its end.

Joni Marie gave me life at the end of hers.

Gazing at the horizon, at the serene white glare in the distance, it reminded me of peace. It reminded me that my mom would tell me she wanted to know who Joni Marie was before she knew who Joni Marie was. My mom wanted to thank her for giving me another life.

Flying close enough to touch the face of the angels that my mom and Joni Marie had become, I suddenly became cognizant of this fact:

My mother gave me my first breath. Joni Marie gave me my second.

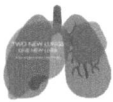

As I take a deep breath now. As I fill my lungs with life given to me. Times two.

#40 – February 6, 2019

When I talk to people about my transplant experience, my favorite topic is how I set out to find people who knew my angel donor, Joni Marie. People who worked with her. I wanted to know more about this generous angel who checked the box to provide me with another life. With a second chance.

I had already been in communication with Joni's mother, and was preparing to visit her shortly. Based on the brief conversations I had with her, I knew my angel donor was a loving mother of two young children, and a beloved daughter. The next step to discover further about this beautiful lady, who I was never supposed to ever cross paths with, was to somehow locate and talk to her co-workers.

Facebook was my tool.

After identifying Joni Marie's parents on that site, I was able to locate the account of my angel donor. Attached to her profile were her last two employers. My angel donor's most recent employer has since gone out of business, which led me to transition to the company where she seemed to be employed prior. Joni Marie's profile showcased her wearing a sweater displaying the logo of that company, where she was pegged to have been a manager.

Although my angel donor's profile did not include where she held that job, I found that company had a location in Joni Marie's hometown. Taking a chance, desiring to walk the floor of where my donor may have walked, I drove to that location.

Securing a parking spot in front of the store, in an area where I could clearly see one of the entrances, I entertained the thought that Joni Marie may have walked through that door daily. That may, in fact, have been the door where she crossed the threshold on her last day there, not imagining someone who was now living because she is no longer, might be observing that same doorway.

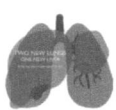

I was determined to enter the store, even though I had no idea whether my angle donor had actually worked there in the past. But I felt my quest to know Joni Marie would not be complete unless I were to speak with someone who worked with her.

In the back of my mind, that was an unattainable desire. After all, this may not even be the location where she worked. And even if this did happen to be her former store, I recognized that someone would have to be in that store, on that day I was visiting, who worked there in 2013, which was the year Joni Marie posted her photo sporting her work sweater.

Confident that it was wholly unrealistic to expect to find an individual who was once a co-worker of my angel donor, I exited my car and walked into the store. I viewed the aisles, I gazed at the displays. Where Joni Marie may have walked, may have organized. At each step, I glanced down at my path, pondering if she had walked that same aisle. If my footsteps matched hers.

During my journey in that space, I passed employees, allowing myself to fantasize that perhaps the man, the woman wearing the company-red polo shirt may have worked with my angel donor. However, each time that idea passed through my mind, I would summarily dismiss it. The possibility seemed entirely faint that I was both in the correct store and that I would find someone who had worked with Joni Marie some five years ago. And I continued my walk.

Until I came to a location in the store that was transformed into a section celebrating the holidays. This is where I viewed a lady constructing a Christmas display. Something pressed me to ask her. That maybe, possibly, this lady could have worked with my angel donor. How could that be, I quizzed myself.

Maybe this was not even Joni Marie's store. How slim the chances were that this particular lady would have worked with her several years ago, even if this did happen to be her store.

Regardless, the voice inside me told me to ask this lady. So, I did.

I slowly approached her and asked if Joni Marie worked there. After displaying a confused and absolutely confounded look for several seconds, she responded that Joni Marie had been dead for two years.

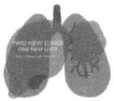

She wanted to know why I asked. Doubting that I should reveal the true cause of my quest, I simply responded that I understood she was an organ donor.

I thanked her and began to turn away, but reversed, asking her what Joni Marie was like. Was she a good person? This lady responded with the statement that Joni Marie was one of her best friends. That Joni Marie had two young children.

That Joni Marie believed deeply in organ donation.

Again, I thanked this lady, began to turn away once more, but reversed again. I turned back to see the lady who considered Joni Marie, my angel donor, to be one of her best friends, on the verge of becoming emotional. I asked the lady her name, and she provided me with it. I then turned away for the final time.

I felt that I had just experienced one of the most magical days of my life. I located where Joni Marie worked. I conversed with a lady who had a shared a strong friendship with Joni Marie, my angel donor.

I told myself that the possibilities of this happening were one in a million.

At the same time, it was that same and identical one in a million possibility that allowed the match that resulted in Joni Marie and me crossing paths nearly 18 months ago. At the end of her life, awarding me with another.

A one in a million chance. A one in a million donor. A one in a million blessing.

#41 – February 18, 2019

Subsequent to the transplant of a fresh pair of lungs and liver from my angel donor during the summer of 2017, I immediately desired to know who my donor was. I yearned to know all about the angel who gave me a fresh start in life. The life that I apparently nearly lost. I also knew the only way to find out was to locate and communicate with my donor's family.

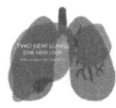

As I was confined to the hospital bed, with a breathing tube placed down my throat, four draining tubes inserted into my chest and sides, hooked up to beeping and monitoring machine after machine, I began to develop in my mind sundry facts I wanted to inquire about from the family of my angel. Who was my donor? What did he or she do? How did he or she pass? How old was this person? Did this person have a family? So much unknown. So many questions.

I was told that once the one-year anniversary of the transplant had passed, I could write a letter to the family, in hopes that they would respond to me. Accordingly, seven days following the first anniversary, on September 1st, just days prior to my 46th birthday, which I nearly did not experience, write that letter I did.

Initially it was difficult to compose the lengthy note. My intent was to pen my thoughts to this person's family, who I didn't know. To a family who tragically lost their mother/daughter/wife/sister unknown to me to some horrible circumstance out of their control. A circumstance that I was totally unaware of. Would they even want to hear from me? Was a year post the turmoil that ended their loved one's life too soon for me to expect them to want to communicate with the person who took the organs of their family member?

Would they be hurt that I was using the life of their precious baby to enjoy my life again, and to do things I never thought I could do anymore? To do things their mother/daughter/wife/sister could never do anymore?

A couple of hours and three and a half pages later, I scrawled out on my laptop the text of my journey for them. My life of Cystic Fibrosis to them. Some of my challenges, my obstacles, my victories. From birth until the age of 44 when I received my angel donor's lungs and liver. And my thankfulness and gratitude since.

And I sent the letter. Unaware of the response I would receive. If I would even receive one. Several weeks later, I did.

The letter was from my donor angel's parents, and I finally learned that the name of the one who gave me that second chance is Joni Marie. That she had two young children left behind. The letter was surely heartfelt and moving.

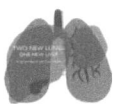

The parents were proud of what their beautiful daughter had done, restoring my life once hers had ended. Among other pearls of facts and feelings shared on that letter, the correspondence informed me that they had previously lost their older daughter 22 years ago, at the age of 44. I found this to be stunning, as I was 44 when Joni Marie, the second daughter they lost, provided me with the invaluable gifts that she did.

Among the details in the letter that I found particularly astounding is the time and date of when Joni Marie's mother was writing the letter. The letter was being written on October 24th, in the 3:00 am hour. Striking to me is that on that same October 24th, and in that same 3:00 am hour, but five time zones to the west, my mother had passed away.

At the identical time my angel donor's mother was composing her innermost thoughts and feelings about her hero daughter whom she lost too soon, my brother and I were at my mom's bedside, thousands of miles away, just hours away from losing our mom too soon.

As some may say, there are no coincidences. That nothing happens by accident. With that, I cannot help but wonder how I was so fortunate to have my life blended with not only a heroic and amazing donor named Joni Marie, but also be bound forever to a such a tender-hearted and giving family, anxious to welcome me as a son into their family.

This occurrence is merely a one in a million chance. A one in a million donor. A one in a million family. A one in a million blessing. And for which I could not be more fortunate.

#42 – February 22, 2019

*A*ny patient with a chronic ailment is uniquely aware that there may come a time. A time when regardless of what is performed, no matter how well attempts to sustain are enacted, despite all best efforts, there may come a time when it all just is not enough.

I recall talking to friends, to co-workers, about the hospitalizations I was undergoing from time to time with my original lungs. Like any

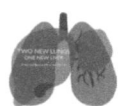

patient with Cystic Fibrosis, as time goes on and as the years pass, the lungs become more and more susceptible to infections. Those infections inevitably lead to hospitalizations and IV treatments. So much so, they are routinely anticipated.

There are points when those two- or three-week reprieves are welcomed. You cling to the expectation that the next treatment will do it. You hope beyond hope that the next iteration of meds will progress you to the stage where you expect the best outcome. The best outcome is a lengthy period away from the hospital and IVs.

The untouchable hope that the next intensive treatment will occur as far in the future as 18 months, as opposed to the typical 12. Or 6. The hope that you never allow yourself to admit is merely a mystical aspiration.

I specifically recall talking to a friend in the secure space of the 19th floor restroom at my workplace many times and several months before my transplant. Our dialogues would center on how I was feeling before and after the hospitalizations and the IVs.

My descriptions would point to a cushion. It was that cushion which is as abstract as a divine nighttime dream, yet equally as invaluable. It was that cushion which drives the wish of healing. The cushion which, when carefully cultivated and managed, can allow one a sense of invulnerability.

While I was vastly, and maybe impractically, confident at all times in my ability to recover from the several and increasingly frequent med treatments, I would tell that particular friend the theory holds that at each time a person undergoes a hospitalization or an IV treatment, the lung function improves, but it never returns to the original state. But that it was okay in my circumstance, because I had enough cushion. As long as I maintained adequate cushion, all would be fine.

I remember telling him there may be a point when I cannot recover my lung function, despite all efforts. Maybe one day.

And I specifically remember disclosing in one conversation, on one day in mid-2017, that I believed I had perhaps reached that point. I thought I may have finally encountered that one day.

Invulnerability remains until reality emerges into a clearer focus.

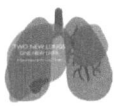

In August 2017, the hospitalizations and IV treatments over my 44 years of life characterized the state of my cushion at the time. The average Lung Allocation Score, a score that estimates the survival rate for those awaiting a lung transplant at a major transplant hospital in the U.S. is 34.5.

My Lung Allocation Score when I was placed onto the transplant list was measured at 43.69. My cushion was evidently close to being exhausted. At the last week of that August, my angel donor, Joni Marie, gave me what no medication could. She allowed me the precious gift of her lungs. Joni Marie not only returned my cushion to me, but her lungs provided me with a fresh cushion. She gave me a re-set. My angel donor took my lung function from 17% pre-transplant to just above 80% approximately a year later.

There are many things for which I thank Joni Marie on a daily basis related to the gifts she unselfishly provided. She gave me a future, when my present was in doubt. She gave me hope, when doubt had become the villain I constantly endeavored to vanquish.

My dreams. My life. All bundled in a cushion of breath. Joni Marie returned that to me. All part of the intangible cushion.

#43 – February 25, 2019

*E*ighteen months ago this morning, I received the call that a donor had become available to provide me with fresh lungs and a liver.

My donor, Joni Marie, gave me the greatest gift of all - a future of a longer and better quality of life. I could not be more grateful for that precious gift. At the same time, I greatly mourn the donor family's loss of their loved one.

Joni Marie has two small children. This past Valentine's Day was the second time their mother was not with them. Joni Marie's children had no mother to which they could present those tiny, colorful heart shaped candies. No notes of love in their very best, practiced handwriting to their mother this year.

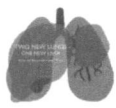

No mother to kiss, hug and tell that they loved her on that special day. No mother to share those affections with again. Not on that day. Not ever.

That family will forever be minus one.

Please consider becoming an organ donor. As of 9:42 am EST today, there are 74,418 individuals who are active waiting list candidates. One person is added to the national transplant waiting list every ten minutes, and in 2017, an average of 18 people died every day while awaiting a transplant.

In 2018, greater than 36,500 transplants, more transplants than ever, were performed. In fact, 2018 was the 6th consecutive record-breaking year.

One donor can save eight lives and affect the lives of countless others. Every life saved creates a story for that person rescued. Take the opportunity to create eight stories.

Take the opportunity to become an everlasting hero to those eight people and to the countless others who they will touch in their lifetime. Their lifetime which would be extended as a result of your unselfish and unending generosity.

It costs nothing to save a life. Live on through others and become that lifelong hero to many.

#44 – February 28, 2019

The other day at the gym, in the early morning hours, I was talking to a gentleman of an older age. I had seen him working out in the past, periodically, from time to time. Another member of the dedicated 4:00 am wake-up team. Always at the machines, lifting and pressing weights likely heavier than my entire body weight, in a repetitive and deliberate manner.

As I transitioned between benches on the far-left corner of the facility, this man flagged me down. He had noticed how I would frequent the gym each day and at the same time. As we talked, he would eye

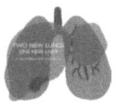

my dark brown cane propped conspicuously against the off-white wall behind the expansive metal weight rack.

During our conversation, I explained that I had a double lung and liver transplant performed about 18 months ago. That it, and the fact that I have Multiple Sclerosis (the reason for the cane, as I informed him), are the reasons I need to exercise each day, and have been since last July, in order to keep my newly rejuvenated health and body in proper working order.

As our dialogue progressed, this man commented that in a matter of the past month and a half since he noticed my attendance at the gym, he felt that I appeared 150% better now than when he first remembered seeing me. Better in my dexterity. In my mobility. In my general composure.

I proceeded to share with him that I owed it all to my angel donor. How she is the one who provided me with a new beginning. With a new ability to live. With a new availability to actively participate in life.

I recalled to myself how, prior to the transplant, although challenged with the occasional need for an oxygen concentrator, I would put aside the nasal cannula for a bit to initiate a clipped workout at home. The attempt to use my couch, with the usage of a cushion, to mimic an incline bench, I would struggle to lift the two five-pound dumbbells I maintained in my apartment. Challenged by both the lack of oxygen and greatly curbed muscular strength, I envisioned my times of weight-lifting were far behind me.

However, as it stands, another gift provided to me by my beautiful angel donor, Joni Marie, is the ability allow myself, through exercise, to preserve the magnificent organs which I have been gifted. Never before had I seen the art of exercise as such a blessing until it was taken from me.

Further, through the dialogue with that fellow gym rat, I was able to share a bit of the story of Joni Marie, my remarkable angel donor. So, an additional person will know what Joni did for me. How Joni has restored my life.

And maybe as a result, a seed will be planted in another's consciousness to remember Joni Marie. To prolong her spirit. To perhaps

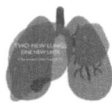

enable another Joni Marie to be a hero to others unknown in future years. To bring about a multitude of further stories to enable new lives and second chances that would have otherwise been lost.

#45 – March 5, 2019

*W*hen someone is born with a condition, a disease, that is deemed to be fatal by all accounts. That is deemed to be fatal by all accounts. By the doctors. By the community. By the family. And eventually by the individual. This is the life of someone with Cystic Fibrosis.

But when this someone receives a lung transplant, it is with the intent of the past forever changing. Evolving into an existence of something glorious.

As if life the patient has previously known it to be is exterminated. Vanished and conquered.

Gone would be the two, three or four-times daily pulmonary treatments at home that never fail to break up your day. No more hospitalizations that never fail to break up your life. All because you would now have lungs that are anticipated to never fail.

The heartbreak occurs when those expectations are not met.

The body is fickle, in that it is forever attempting to reject the new organs that have been gifted. The promised bulwark against that threat is a life-long cocktail of anti-rejection pills and vitamins awarded to the transplantee. This shield holds the dream of an extended life, free from the suffering and inconveniences to which the Cystic has become accustomed.

The heartbreak occurs when those expectations are not met.

Subsequent to the transplant, the cylindrical, dark green metal oxygen tank is placed into a closet. The nebulizer is tucked away deep into a drawer. The Vest machine is placed in the attic. All past lifesaving aids are barred into the deepest cervices of the mind, never to be resurrected because fresh lungs have now been securely positioned and emplaced.

The heartbreak occurs when those expectations are not met.

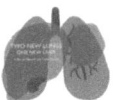

The photo of a Vest machine sitting in a garage belonging to a little girl from Virginia who was granted her wings as a CF Angel due to complications maybe a year after her lung transplant.

The story told by a lady in Texas who had a little sister with CF, who left her two years post-transplant following a six-month battle with the new lungs.

The Facebook message from a brave and strong CFer in Illinois who received new lungs a year and a half ago. This young lady who has been in the hospital for over a week and is again connected to oxygen assistance. Ever positive, as only a battle-tested CF Warrior could be, she states toward the end of her posting, "I never thought I'd be back here again."

The heartbreak occurs when those expectations are not met.

#46 – March 16, 2019

It was the day. The day I never imagined would ever be. The day I had been proclaiming to all who questioned that I did not need. That despite my having Cystic Fibrosis, 17% lung function and oxygen assistance, in my mind, I was a type of Superman who did not and would not ever need a lung transplant.

As sure as the world spins and the tides rise and fall, my plane was leaving for Dallas late that summer afternoon, ultimately leading to an admission to University of Texas Southwestern to be placed onto the list for a lung and liver transplant upon arrival on the continent.

It would not be truthful or accurate to surmise that I was scared about possibly undergoing a potentially half-day procedure where my damaged and scarred organs would be substituted with healthy replacements from an unknown angel donor at some point. I was merely checking the box to have something executed which I knew, as sure as I was breathless, would never occur because 1) an appropriate donor would never be found in time and 2) if a donor was found, the fresh lungs and liver would not be adequate for me – and I would be woken up and sent home.

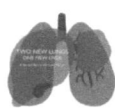

Oddly enough, none of that bothered me. I firmly believed I was going to live longer than Moses.

By traveling to this transplant center, I was merely checking the box.

Before I left my place, knowing I would not see it again for some time, I glanced about the living area of my one room dwelling that was cluttered with used Kleenexes. Two trash cans brimming with them, allowing the contents to spill onto the dusty, cherry-red laminate flooring. Tissues containing, with each cough, the remnants of lungs with steadily declining functionality, with those failing keepers of oxygen acting as an undesired and endless expectorant.

I was thankful to have made arrangements with a good friend to transport me to the airport. I was worried that an Uber or a Lyft driver would deny me any transport, given my physical appearance at that stage – pale, thin, weak, coughing. Sickly.

A secondary concern of mine would be that I could pass out from a lack of oxygen on the way to the airport, and doing so in a ride-sharing vehicle would not be my preferred option. This was a far-fetched possibility, but one that I hesitantly allowed to enter the edges of my thoughts far too often.

This was a new part of my journey. A journey I never wanted. A journey I never expected. But a journey to a potential new life.

Attached to a portable oxygen concentrator, wheeled to the First-Class section of the 767-100, I settled into my spacious seat. With this being the first step to what could be my new life, I desired to spend the next five hours with an extra eight inches of leg room that only elite accommodations could offer.

As the plane lifted off into the afternoon sky over Hawaii en route to the mainland, I questioned myself rhetorically. Would I return home to Hawaii with new lungs in three months? Would I come back in nine months? Would I ever come back to Hawaii? Would this be my last plane flight ever?

All of that was secondary to whether I would live long enough for a donor to be found once I reached Dallas. Time would be the moderator to adjudicate that decision.

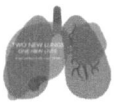

Oddly enough, none of that bothered me. I firmly believed I was going to live longer than Moses.

By traveling to this transplant center, I was merely checking the box.

On the morning of August 25, 2017, I received a call that my angel donor had been found. It had been decided that Joni Marie would be my angel donor.

She checked the box.

Within a couple of days, I took my first breath with my new lungs. With Joni Marie's lungs. The lungs of an angel.

The lungs I never wanted. The lungs I never expected. But these are the lungs of Joni Marie. The lungs that I will never live without.

#47 – March 17, 2019

This afternoon, I shared with a neighbor the beautiful story of my donor and my path to know her after the transplant.

The story started with a picture of Joni Marie, my angel donor.

The story continued with how I wrote to and communicated with my donor's family. How I drove to meet her parents a few states north. How I visited my donor's house. How I discovered and traveled to my donor's previous workplace. How I happened upon a former colleague at her store who proclaimed to me that my donor was one of her best friends. How I believed Joni Marie directed me to her best friend.

It is the special story, the beauty of a relationship of those who receive organs in their time of need from angel donors. A story when ordinary people become heroes when acting upon the seemingly inconsequential decision to check a box. A box printed on a plain, ivory sheet of paper. The image of an empty square floating on the liquid crystal display of a laptop.

That is a box of life.

That two-dimensional box provides hope of many dimensions.

It represents the hope of the person who is donating organs. The hope that they will live on.

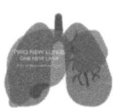

The hope that what they have accomplished in life will not end but will rather continue in another's life; the life of another whose existence would have ceased in an untimely and cruel manner before their dreams, wishes, and goals were fulfilled.

It represents the hope of the person who is receiving the organs. The hope that they will live on.

The hope that perhaps a life that, from an early age, the person did not expect to last. The hope that they will be able to graduate from high school. The hope that they might meet a special somebody one day, fall in love, and get married.

The hope that they will celebrate with their daughter who has met a perfect gentleman and will be able to dance the final time with their little girl, as daddy's princess begins an enchanted new life.

The hope that this time they are holding their husband's hand before the attendee whisks them into the cold, sterile operating room will not be the last.

There is a magic in that hope. There is a purpose beyond our time on this earth. The purpose is to continue, extend, and expand life beyond our own. That begins with checking a box.

That is a box of life.

That two-dimensional box provides hope of many dimensions.

My beautiful angel donor, Joni Marie, checked that box.

My beautiful angel donor, Joni Marie, continued, extended and expanded my life beyond her own.

This afternoon, I shared with a neighbor the beautiful story of my donor and my path to getting to know her after the transplant.

The story started with a picture of Joni Marie, my angel donor.

#48 – March 24, 2019

As we progress through life, transitioning through different and various stages, those who are important to us are defined. Perhaps by their humor. Maybe because of their wealth. It could be their charisma that gives them an edge.

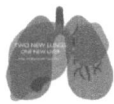

Or possibly it is because they made the extra effort to care for us, and in the end saved our life.

It was some seven years ago at this writing when I was told that there was a Cystic Fibrosis doctor in Hawaii. This was significant, as it had been decades since a certified civilian CF doctor had practiced in the state.

A doctor specializing in CF is one of a kind. Given this, I jumped at the opportunity to become his patient.

At my first appointment with this specialty doctor, my Pulmonary Function Test recorded my lung function at 25%. With my lungs functioning at a quarter of full capacity, it was recommended that I be assessed for a lung transplant at that time. Expecting to live forever, literally, there was not even a mere glimmer of the prospect of me acting on that suggestion. There was no reason for such an invasive, drastic, radical, and in my mind, an unproven, procedure. 25% lung function would serve me adequately for the remainder of my life.

As the years crept forward, the condition of my lungs deteriorated like an aging avocado ravaged by time and faulty genetics. Several infections, hospitalizations and subsequent IV treatments with the most robust drugs geared to torment the several potentially deadly bacteria served to slow the deterioration of my lungs. It did not, however, halt the damage being incurred.

For three of the last eight months prior to being gifted with new lungs, I was interned at Straub Medical Center, shackled to an IV pole housing several bags of medication. Continually dosed with the healing liquid for a good three quarters of each day. Executing heaving coughing fits bringing about near discharge more than once. Expelling two and a half sputum cups of blood at one point.

It was a Tuesday night in mid to late July 2017. I had just finished a hospitalization yet was still not feeling well when I was in my doctor's office one evening after work. He was strongly advising me to leave for the mainland in order to be listed for a double lung and liver transplant. Most tests for the designated hospital in Texas had already been completed, arrangements made, largely through the workings and efforts

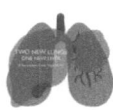

of my doctor. He was ready to press the button that would send me to Dallas, where I could be eligible for the life-saving transplant.

But I was the barrier. 17% lung function. Lips colored with a shade of blue, because I did not feel the necessity to wear oxygen when discussing a need for a transplant with my doctor that night. I did not need a transplant, my inner musings assured me.

I was going to live longer than Moses. A mantra I held onto tightly. I honestly thought I was never going to die. Ever.

From both a professional and personal standpoint, my doctor told me repeatedly that evening I had to leave the island by that weekend, in just a few days, because his concern was that I was rapidly becoming too sick to fly.

If I was to degenerate to that point, I would essentially be stuck. I would not receive a transplant, as Hawaii does not perform lung and liver transplants. I would effectively not live longer than Moses.

The minutes of the dialogue passed. His arguments became more convincing. The reasons for attempting a transplant were providing me with a good basis for giving this procedure a try.

After five years of on and off banter about a transplant, and an hour of pointed and emotional testimony, my doctor won me over. I would be on a plane en route to Dallas in a few days.

Approximately six weeks after that evening conversation in the brightly lit room of my doctor's office on Keeaumoku Street, my angel donor, Joni Marie, was located. Tragedy had fallen upon her. Due to her generosity and foresight, Joni Marie provided me with her physical soul at the end of her physical days.

On August 25, 2017, two people became personally deemed as among the most important people in my life. My angel donor for giving me another chance. And my physician, Dr. Wu, for convincing me with his heartfelt plea to board that plane in late July, and to take that first step toward Joni Marie.

It is thanks to those two that I am breathing, and that I am alive to type the last sentence of this post.

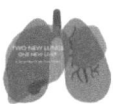

#49 – March 24, 2019

It was nineteen months ago today, perhaps even nineteen months ago at this moment of writing, when I was living in a motel room in Dallas, Texas with 17% lung function. Trying to keep my oxygen saturation level above 88% so I would not have to again loop the tubing around and above my ears and fit the nasal cannula against my upper lip in order to keep from becoming lightheaded. Coughing and hoping there would be no blood product in my sputum, as that could foretell greater damage to my already battered and worn lungs.

It was nineteen months ago today, perhaps even nineteen months ago at this moment of writing, when I knew that would be unacceptable, as I was hoping for a donor, hoping a lung and liver donor could be located, to provide me with a second chance at life. Further damage to my lungs would accelerate the pace of that stubbornly ticking clock. That ticking clock which contained the alarm each and every Cystic Fibrosis patient has been told about his or her entire life. The alarm the CF patient is aware of. Is aware of and never wants to hear but knows it will be sounded someday, any day, too soon.

The alarm which has the bell that cannot be un-rung.

It was nineteen months ago today, perhaps even nineteen months ago at this moment of writing, when in a brightly lit room, surrounded by monitors, insistently beeping monitors, in a North Dallas hospital, the family of my angel donor, Joni Marie, was with their beautiful daughter. Their beautiful daughter who had two young children who loved their mother more than anything. Their beautiful daughter who would do and did anything to please her young children. Their beautiful daughter who was about to cross the boundary. To cross and enter the other side.

It was nineteen months ago today, perhaps even nineteen months ago at this moment of writing, when I was in a motel room, contemplating whether a qualified donor with healthy and clean lungs and liver would ever be found. Concurrently, I was aware of and appreciated that each additional day I waited, my unidentified donor would be spending an additional day with his or her loved ones. Not knowing that that additional day would be their last.

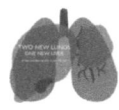

It was nineteen months ago today, perhaps even nineteen months ago at this moment of writing, when I was unaware that the following day would be the first day of the rest of my life.

#50 – March 25, 2019

Nineteen months ago this morning, I received the call that a donor had become available to provide me with fresh lungs and a liver.

My donor, Joni Marie, gave me the greatest gift of all - a future of a longer and better quality of life. I could not be more grateful for that precious gift. At the same time, I greatly mourn the donor family's loss of their loved one.

Joni Marie has two small children who have experienced their second winter without their mother. They missed enjoying their first snowfall with their mother. They missed spending Christmas with their mother. They missed celebrating a New Year with their mother.

As a new season approaches, this is now the second year that Joni Marie's children will miss sharing in the wonderment and beauty of spring flowers with her.

That family will forever be minus one.

Please consider becoming an organ donor. As of 4:50 am EST today, there are 74,490 individuals who are active waiting list candidates. One person is added to the national transplant waiting list every ten minutes, and in 2017, an average of 18 people died every day while awaiting a transplant.

In 2018, greater than 36,500 transplants, more transplants than ever, were performed. In fact, 2018 was the 6th consecutive record-breaking year.

One donor can save eight lives and affect the lives of countless others. Every life saved creates a story for that person rescued. Take the opportunity to create eight stories.

Take the opportunity to become an everlasting hero to those eight people and to the countless others who they will touch in their lifetime.

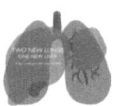

Their lifetime which would be extended as a result of your unselfish and unending generosity.

It costs nothing to save a life. Live on through others and become that lifelong hero to many.

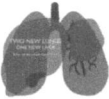